Preventing and Controlling Burnout!

Control Excess Stress for a Healthier and Happier Life

RON KNESS

Contents

Disclaimer

This publication is for informational purposes only and is not intended as medical advice. Medical advice should always be obtained from a qualified medical professional for any health conditions or symptoms associated with them.

Every possible effort has been made in preparing and researching this material. We make no warranties with respect to the accuracy, applicability of its contents or any omissions.

See your healthcare professional before starting any diet or exercise program!

Introduction: What Is Burnout?

Are you "burned out"? If so, you probably understand the definition of this phrase quite well. But just for fun, let's take a look at how that term is defined, and where it originated. As far as definitions go, a burnout is a:

> 1 – reduction of a fuel or substance to nothing, through use or combustion.

> 2 – physical or mental collapse caused by overwork or stress.

You are no doubt familiar with that second definition as it relates to people. It clearly expresses the dangerous repercussions of overwork or stress, when it leads to total collapse or incapacitation of the mind and/or body.

However, that first definition is important to note as well. When you suffer from burnout, you have run out of fuel. You have no energy. You are totally "used up". When a fire runs out of oxygen and combustible material, it 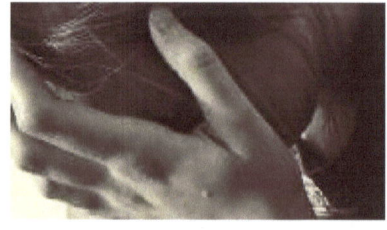 dies. When an engine of any kind has no more fuel, it stops working. These were the types of scenarios that led American psychologist Dr. Herbert Freudenberger to coin the term "burnout" in the 1970s.

He noticed nurses, doctors and other health care providers working endlessly to help others. Many of them often sacrificed their own health, both mental and physical, to help their patients enjoy a better standard of living. These caring individuals were so laser focused on creating positive change in the lives of others that they ignored their own needs.

This led to chronic exhaustion, listlessness, and an in capability to cope with normal, everyday situations. These people were literally "burned out".

These days the term burnout can refer to anyone. It is not just health care providers that can totally overwork themselves to the point of absolute exhaustion. The problem is that psychological and medical authorities have not come up with a concrete definition that gives us a word-by-word description of burnout. This lack of agreement nationally and globally on exactly what constitutes a burned out individual means that we don't understand the commonality of this debilitating situation.

Suffice it to say that burnout can be considered much different than mere stress. It is like stress on steroids. Suffer enough chronic stress without being treated properly, and you could end up burned out. What is the difference between burnout and stress? Let's take a look.

Stress Verses Burnout: What's the Difference?

Did you know that some stress is actually good for you? Seriously, you would literally not be able to survive some situations if your body did not know how to respond to stress. If your entire life is sunshine and roses, and you never experience negative emotions or situations of any kind, you would be totally unprepared for your first encounter with stress. There is no doubt though that chronic stress can be harmful. It can actually damage your immune system, leading to a heightened chance of falling prey to disease, sickness and illness.

On the other hand, there are good types of stress as well. Firdaus Dhabhar, PhD, is an Associate Professor of Psychiatry and Behavioral Sciences at the Stanford Center on Stress and Health, reminds us that short-term stress is actually beneficial, when it is not recurring or chronic. When you encounter stress for just a few minutes, or even an hour, your fight or flight response is triggered.

When this happens, the hormonal and chemical calls to action in your body are positive. You are highly alert and aware. All your senses come alive. Your brain function improves substantially. You have detected stress of some kind, so your immune system immediately responds.

There are studies which show that this type of short-term stress can instantly improve your body's natural defense system, and help you ward off disease and infection.

Now imagine that situation over the long term. Your senses are hyper-alert for days, weeks and months, instead of just a few minutes or hours at a time. There are no significant rest periods between your stressful states. This is when stress leads to burnout.

Short-term, acute periods of stress are normal and actually benefit your body and your mind. They teach you how to deal with future stress, and trigger your survival instincts. Without this type of short-term 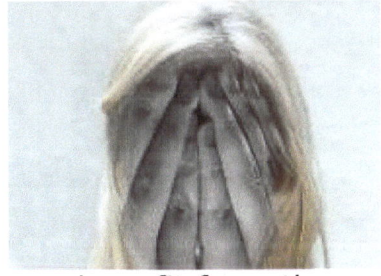 stress, a hungry lion would never benefit from the boost of physical and mental energy required to chase down an antelope.

That same antelope would alternately never have a chance of escape, if stress didn't trigger the appropriate response. On the other hand, once your systems can no longer deal with stress because it is a constant presence in your life, your body and mind give out.

This certainly doesn't mean you should seek out stressful situations. The typical human encounters several short-term stress-triggers every day.

You are running late for work. You didn't receive a return phone call you have been expecting. You get a letter in the mail that does not deliver good news.

Speaking of news, media outlets online, in print and on television make sure that you have plenty to be stressed out about. Don't actively seek stress if you are generally stress-free. You will experience short-term stress soon enough.

How Burnout Affects You

You just learned, possibly for the first time, that short-term periods of stress are beneficial. As long as you have sufficient periods of no stress between your short-term stress triggers, your body and mind benefit. Continual, ever-present stress leads to burnout. Unfortunately, many burned-out individuals never recover completely from the situation. That is why it is so important to constantly monitor your environment and relationships, so you can avoid burnout altogether.

Studies on brain chemistry show that burnout can cause long-lasting neurological problems. Your brain controls everything you do. Your brain is crucial for normal bodily function, and is the core of what allows you to exist. A normally functioning brain is so important to human survival that a lack of brainwave activity is one of the requirements for a declaration of death.

Burnout can cause negative changes in your brain chemistry that, if left untreated, can do lifelong damage.

Several studies have been conducted to show just how a burned out brain is affected. Doctor Armita Golkar led one particular study that was held at the Karolinska Institute in Sweden.

It has been cited by the Association of Psychological Science as important for understanding the chronic stress/brain connection. Basically, the findings showed that burnout actually changes *"neural circuits in the brain and hurts people's ability to cope with stressful situations."*

This means that a terribly vicious cycle develops.

The more stressed you are on a consistent basis, the harder it is for you to deal with stressful situations in the future. This affects your neural circuitry negatively, further weakening a healthy stress response. So any future stress becomes harder and harder to deal with, even if it would not be particularly stressful for a healthy brain. The cycle continues to the point where just about anything causes stress, and the sufferer of this condition cannot function normally.

Doctor Golkar tested 40 volunteers that had been diagnosed with burnout syndrome (more on the signs and symptoms of burnout in the next section). These particular participants all blamed their conditions on work-related stress that was ever-present and ongoing. They worked 60, 70 or more hours every week, continuously, for many years. Also in the study were 70 healthy, "burnout free" volunteers with no history of chronic stress.

All 110 subjects were asked to view pictures which typically caused negative or neutral emotional responses. However they responded on a per-picture basis, the participants were asked to maintain, suppress or intensify their emotional response. While the volunteers were focusing on the pictures being shown as well as their emotional responses, a loud, startling sound interrupted their concentration.

Those individuals diagnosed with burnout had a much more difficult time suppressing their reactions to the loud noise. Across the board, the results were the same. This led Doctor Golkar to hypothesize that a brain which has already been chronically stressed to the point of burnout has a much more difficult time dealing with new stressors than a healthy brain. The test subjects which did not suffer from burnout were able to control their responses to the interrupting noise much more effectively than their burned-out counterparts.

All participants were also given brain scans while they were simply sitting quietly.

The stressed-out participants, as a whole, showed significantly larger amygdalas. This is the area of the brain which is associated with aggression and fear. Not only was the amygdala larger and thus more ready to attach stress to any situation or event, but the connection between the amygdala and medial prefrontal cortex was much weaker than in the healthy brains.

Your medial prefrontal cortex is the part of your brain related to executive function. These are mental skills that help you accomplish certain tasks. Executive function allows you to easily switch your focus from one task, activity or thought to another. When healthy, it allows you to remember details, plan and organize, and manage your time.

When unhealthy you can't pay attention, you consistently say or do the wrong thing in a certain situation, and you forget what your experiences have taught you in the past. This shows undeniably that burnout leads to a reduced ability to deal with stress in the future, and also negatively affects your ability to make simple decisions and perform simple actions.

Aside from this mental damage, burnout can literally change your body, and not in a good way.

When you suffer from burnout, you have very little to no mental and physical energy. This leads to little physical activity. Your body begins to atrophy, from head to toe. Your body is also negatively affected because of your weakened immune system. Your natural immunity is your body's defense system against illness, disease and infection.

As mentioned previously, an individual diagnosed with burnout has a lowered immunity to infection and disease than normal.

This means a burned out individual is more likely to succumb to disease, illness and sickness which creates negative changes in your body. Let's take a look at how to identify burnout, so you can seek treatment as quickly as possible.

The Signs and Symptoms of Burnout

As with any health condition, there are certain signs that indicate burnout is present, or right around the corner. If you can identify with more than 2 or 3 of the following burnout symptoms, you should consider scheduling an appointment with your doctor for a professional diagnosis.

- Feel alone in the world, helpless, defeated and "trapped"

- Suffer from frequent headaches, muscle aches and back pain

- Withdraw from responsibilities

- Loss of motivation, you just don't care

- Feeling tired, exhausted and "drained" most of the time

- A cynical or negative outlook that gets increasingly worse

- Are constantly sick (sign of a weak immune system)

- Self-medicating with alcohol, food and/or drugs

- Never happy, and nothing you do is ever good enough

- A constant sense of self-doubt and failure

- A recent and drastic change in sleep habits and/or appetite

- Withdraw from society

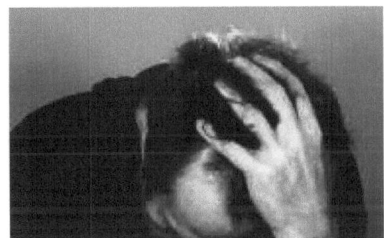

What Causes Burnout?

Now that you know the warning signs of burnout, what causes it? Are there specific circumstances or activities which increase your chance of becoming burned out? Every human being is different. So sometimes, what could cause one person chronic stress that leads to burnout could be a situation which doesn't affect someone else negatively at all.

However, in general you should be aware of the following scenarios and stressors which increase the possibility of becoming a burned out individual.

Lack of control – When you feel like you have no control over your life, you are experiencing a stressful situation.

Constant overwork – You need balance in your life. Constantly being overworked and over-stressed, in your career or personal life, can lead to burnout.

You don't feel satisfied or rewarded – This includes feelings of under-appreciation at work, and in your personal life.

You don't feel a sense of community or belonging – When you feel like you're the only person on the outside looking in, this is a very lonely, stressful experience.

A constant presence of conflicting values –
People do not perform well when they are constantly
surrounded by situations, events and people that
conflict with their personal set of values.

You feel unfairly treated – When you perceive
that everyone is getting a "fairer shake" than you,
this could lead to chronic stress and burnout.

**Spending all of your time accomplishing tasks
and taking care of responsibilities, and no time
enjoying life and its many rewards –** This one is
self-explanatory.

Remember, the causes of stress in your life may be
different from someone else. Basically, anything that
makes you feel emotionally drained, overwhelmed
and unable to the degree where you cannot meet the
demands of daily life could be steering you down the
path to burnout.

9-Step Plan to Deal With Burnout

Obviously, avoiding burnout is your best case scenario. Once you have been diagnosed with burnout syndrome, there are steps you should take as well. The following steps will help you prevent from getting burned out, and also help you deal with burnout if you already suffer from this condition.

1 – Get Moving

Physical movement leads to so many health benefits. It keeps your brain alert, boosts your heart health, and ramps up your natural ability to resist infection and disease. Your physical body, inside and out, becomes stronger and healthier. Your organs and all of the interior processes which allow you to function and exist also become healthier.

Don't worry, you won't have to purchase an expensive gym or health club membership. You also don't have to transform from the couch potato to Olympic athlete overnight either.

Look at opportunities every day to stand up as opposed to sitting down. Take the stairs instead of the elevator, and park further away from your work entrance than you usually do. Spend part of your lunch break walking, and engage in some type of aerobic activity at least 3 times a week.

The key here is to get more physical movement and exercise into your life. You benefit is overall health and well-being, and exercise acts like a wonder drug to prevent and treat burnout.

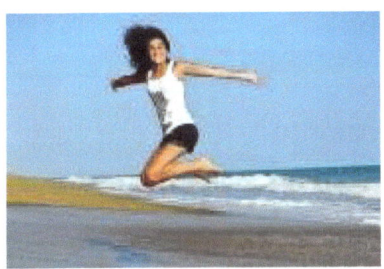

2 – Get Enough Rest

Physical activity is important to beat stress and keep burnout at bay, but rest is just as important. Adults need between 7 and 8 hours of restful sleep every night. Proper sleep has been linked to dramatically lower levels of stress. Adults who get plenty of rest are also generally healthier overall than their sleep deprived counterparts. Less stress and a healthy body due to proper rest make an effective tool for burnout prevention and treatment.

3 – Eat Smart

Nutritionists now believe that is much as 60% to 75% of your level of fitness and health is due to your diet alone. This is why it is so important to monitor what you put into your body.

Less processed foods

If your diet consists mostly of food items that are wrapped, bagged, boxed and canned, you are eating a lot of processed foods that are pumped full of harmful toxins, preservatives, steroids and other unhealthy chemicals and minerals.

Start eating more foods that are as close to their natural state as possible. Switching much of your diet to raw foods has been shown to have immediate health benefits. If eating raw fruits, vegetables, nuts and berries is out of the question for you, you can still cook them. Opt for broiled or steamed over fried, and make sure you're getting wild caught salmon, grass fed beef and organic eggs in your diet as well.

These days there is no excuse for claiming ignorance where diet is concerned. You know you should be eating more fruits and vegetables, and less drive-through and restaurant foods. Doing so reduces your chances of becoming burned out, and has been proven to reduce burnout symptoms in those that have been diagnosed with this condition.

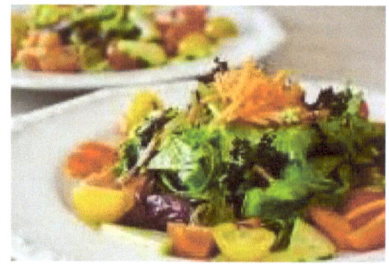

4 – Stay Hydrated

How important is hydration to health? In one of many similar studies, patients suffering from Alzheimer's had their daily water intake raised. Simply increasing the amount of water those Alzheimer's sufferers drank on a daily basis dramatically decreased the debilitating symptoms they were suffering from. This is how crucial water is to overall mental and physical health, and preventing burnout.

The human body can go for 30 or more days without eating any food. However, human beings can't go more than 3 days without drinking water. You do receive some of water in the foods that you eat. However, this is never enough to properly hydrate your body for maximum health benefits. You have probably heard the advice which recommends drinking eight 8-ounce glasses of water a day. It is not an exaggeration; if anything that is a minimum amount of water you should be drinking. This is a good rule of thumb for keeping hydrated.

The thing about drinking water is you really can't overdo yourself, in most cases. Water is an excellent detox agent, flushing your body of dangerous toxins, poisons and waste. When your body is healthy, it deals with stress effectively. As well as preventing burnout, a properly hydrated body has a better chance of coping with burnout than a body that is thirsting for hydration.

5 – Limit Exposure to Triggers

You are probably aware of a few things in your life that cause stress. Limit your exposure to these stressors. Smart dieters trying to lose weight surround themselves with healthy food. They also steer clear of situations where unhealthy food is present. Do the same. Whether you are trying to treat or prevent burnout, staying away from stressful situations in the first place just makes sense.

6 – Socialize for Support

There is a lot of evidence which suggests socialization can reduce stress. When you socialize, you generally "hang out" with people like yourself. This is why animals herd in the wild. There is a feeling of safety in numbers. Sitting at home alone and brooding on your problems is never the right answer. This often leads to blowing your situation out of proportion, and creating more stress than is actually present. Socialization has also proven successful in treating burnout as well as preventing it.

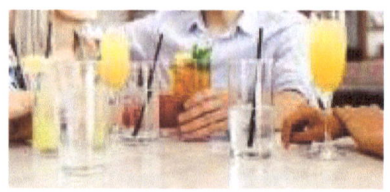

7 – Practice Stress Relief Techniques

You can meditate just about anywhere, at any time you have 5, 10 or 15 spare minutes. Meditation has been used as a calming, stress-relief practice for centuries. Aromatherapy, acupuncture, acupressure, deep breathing and taking frequent work breaks are all effective stress-relief techniques.

8 - Schedule Your Life, But Remain Flexible

When you are unprepared, you are often stressed out. Organize and schedule your life. Create to-do lists and carry a daily planner with you. There is a wonderful sense of control and peace of mind when you make a schedule and stick to it. However, make sure you leave room for flexibility, or an unforeseen conflict with an unforgiving schedule could cause for a stressful situation.

9 – Get Some Sun Every Day

Your body needs a healthy amount of vitamin D to function properly. As mentioned earlier, when your body is healthy and strong, it is easier for you to deal with stress.

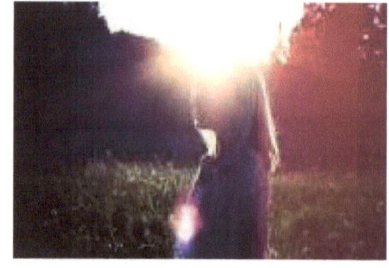

When your skin is exposed to 15 to 20 minutes of sun each day, your body creates the required amount of vitamin D. You should obviously not strip down to your birthday suit, but the more of your skin that absorbs the sun's rays the better for healthy vitamin D production.

Understanding the Difference Between Burnout and Depression

A lot of people who are "burned out" show signs of depression. Depression is often an indicator that someone has a burnout syndrome. What's the difference? These terms are often used interchangeably. However, even though they are related in some ways, they're not actually the same.

Stress has a lot to do with both burnout and depression.

When you are challenged in any way, mentally or physically, emotionally or spiritually, your body releases adrenaline and cortisol. These are known as the "stress hormones". Your pulse quickens, your breathing becomes deep, your heart starts pumping blood at a faster rate. All of your senses are on high alert. This is part of your "fight or flight" response, which has allowed human beings to survive and rule the planet for eons.

Chronic stress, when your body is constantly releasing stress hormones, can lead to a situation where you simply cannot cope with the never-ending stress in your life. When you feel out of control, like there is no end in sight to the turmoil in your life, depression is a normal reaction. Unfortunately, so is burnout when your stress is left untreated.

The Definitions of Burnout and Depression

The **U.S. National Library of Medicine** defines depression as:

"A state of low mood and aversion to activity that can affect a person's thoughts, behavior, feelings and sense of well-being."

That respected health institution goes on to say that depression episodes are short-lived. A constantly depressed state is a sign of possible burnout. The **Mental Health Foundation in the United Kingdom** gives us this depression definition:

"Depression is a common mental disorder that causes people to experience depressed mood, loss of interest or pleasure, feelings of guilt or low self-worth, disturbed sleep or appetite, low energy, and poor concentration."

On the other hand, psychologist Sherrie Bourg Carter of the magazine and website *Psychology Today* tells us that burnout:

"Is more than just a bad day or a bad week. It's a problem that significantly interferes with one's health, happiness, and over quality of life."

She goes on to say the difference between a stressed-out individual experiencing depression, and burnout, "is a matter of degree".

The respected health authority that is the **Mayo Clinic** has this to say about burnout:

"Burnout is a special type of stress – a chronic state of physical, emotional or mental exhaustion."

As you can see, when depression is long-term, it is often a sign of burnout. Many people enter a distressed state of emotions periodically. Put another way, you may be depressed if you experience a bad day from time to time. Your issue might be burnout if you feel that every day is a bad day. If you do feel depressed or stressed out constantly, your issue could be burnout, which can lead to serious health problems long-term when left untreated.

6 Tips for Achieving a Healthy Work/Life Balance

A happy, stress-free, successful life is all about balance. Focus on nothing but your career and climbing the corporate ladder, and you miss out on incredible, once-in-a-lifetime moments with your loved ones. Of course, the opposite is true as well.

If you neglect your career and spend every waking moment concerned about your family and loved ones, you will end up underachieving on the job, and your family will pay the price in the long run.

You have heard the stories from more than one regretful senior citizen. Thinking it was the best thing for his family, a man aggressively sinks all his time and effort into his career so he can make more and more money.

Over the decades he misses his child's first steps, graduations, birthdays and anniversaries, and important "firsts" which cannot be relived. He was successful in his job, providing wealth and stability for his family. However, he was never really part of the family, just that absentee dad and grandfather that paid all the bills.

On the other hand, you could invest all of your energy on spending time with your friends and family members. You use your sick days and personal time at work for ball games, birthdays and other celebrations.

You are never really "present" on the job, so long after you should have been promoted several times, you are still at an entry-level position. Your family suffers mightily where finances and stability are concerned, and your children grow up believing living a stressful paycheck to paycheck existence is acceptable.

If you are seeking a healthy balance in your life in regards to your career and your personal relationships, consider this. The word balance is defined as:

> "*Balance - noun - an even distribution of weight enabling someone or something to remain upright and steady*."

To keep your personal and career lives in balance, keeping every aspect of your life "upright and steady", practice the following 6 tips.

1 – Review Constantly

At work you have performance reviews. Every 30 days, 90 days, semiannually or every year, your supervisor discusses your past performance with you.

This is usually a back-and-forth conversation, where each of you can objectively review your work effort. A very important part of business performance reviews is planning for the future, in order to correct problematic behavior and accidental mistakes, and to keep you on the right path for advancement in the company.

Unfortunately, performance reviews in interpersonal relationships don't happen on a specific schedule. Just as unfortunate is the fact that you will receive criticism and critiques from everyone in your life, whether that person should be a force of influence in planning your behavior and actions or not. To correct this, sit down with your loved ones on a regular basis. Review the relationships you have with your friends and family members.

Don't look at your life through rose-colored glasses. Be honest with yourself. Give, and accept, healthy criticism from the people in your personal life that mean the most to you. Successful relationships are hard work. They take dedication and effort. Review your personal relationships regularly, take action to correct past mistakes, and lay the groundwork for healthy relationships in the future.

2 – Give Yourself a Reward for Working Hard

Money is an unfortunate necessity in life. You must have money to keep a roof over your head, to pay necessary bills, and to feed your family.

That is the reason why the majority of people work. If all of your bills could be taken care of, and you and your family could live comfortably without you working, wouldn't that be great? In other words, people take on jobs and try to advance in their careers so that they can finance a personal life that is attractive to them.

This usually means working hard. However, you can easily suffer "burnout" if you overwork yourself. To keep this from happening, and to keep your personal and career lives balanced, plan down-time in your schedule. Write down weekly, monthly and annual personal-life rewards that you can look forward to.

It is a lot easier to bust your rear-end at work if you see on your calendar at home that you and your family will be enjoying a week-long vacation next month. This gives you something to look forward to and performs as an incentive to keep you on the correct career path, so you can enjoy personal rewards.

3 – Divorce Yourself from the Emotional Vampires in Your Life

One of the hardest things to do in your personal life is to distance yourself from a friend. However, this is sometimes exactly what you must do to create a stable and balanced career/personal life. You may have a friend who constantly brings you down. They always have drama in their life.

It seems like they can't exist unless they are sapping your mental and emotional energy.

Sound familiar?

Start spending less time with this person. Your love for them never needs to wane. However, you are doing them a disservice by enabling this behavior.

You are also creating stress which affects both your job and personal life performances. Instead of interacting with this person on a daily or weekly basis, spend some quality time with them once or twice a month. This will make you appreciate their company more than you currently do, and may help them understand that their behavior needs an adjustment as well.

4 – Exercise

Physical activity leads to improved mental functioning as well as physical health. On the physical side of the equation, a strong, healthy body gives you lots of energy. Whether playing with the grand-kids or working long hours at your job, regular exercise will pay off. With a busy work or personal schedule this means planning ahead.

You should always prioritize those things that are important, and since exercise leads to a healthier mind and body, make sure that you schedule it regularly.

A fit body also leads to a reduced chance of contracting debilitating chronic disease and infection, which helps you in every aspect of your life.

5 – Schedule Relaxing Mini-Breaks

Learn to meditate for 5 or 10 minutes at a time. Spend that same amount of time taking a walk around your house, or outside of your work environment. The key here is to remember that a little relaxation goes a long way towards balance and peace of mind in every aspect of your life. Several times a day you should "check out" mentally and physically.

Sometimes, we become so focused on what we are doing we can't see the forest for the trees. Plan several 5, 10 or 15-minute breaks throughout your day. If you are at work, take this time to call a loved one. On the weekend, when you are spending all of your time with friends and family members, take a few minutes to spend by yourself. These mini-breaks allow you to look at all aspects of your life in an objective manner, and you will sometimes spot opportunities for balancing and out-of-proportion life/career situation.

6 – Plan Short-Term, Mid-term and Long-Term Goals

You would never think about taking a trip without mapping out your journey ahead of time.

This is important in your personal and business lives as well. Set your priorities, writing down specific goals you want to achieve in your personal and career relationships. These should be short-term (30, 60, 90 and 180-day) goals, as well as mid-term (1, 3 and 5-year) and long-term (10, 20, 30-year) targets as well.

Burnout Checklist

Dr. Herbert Freudenberger coined the term "burnout" in the 1970s, to refer to health care providers and professionals that sacrificed their own health and well-being to heal and treat others.

Here are a few key things to know about burnout:

☐ Stress can be defined as a "physical or mental collapse caused by overwork or stress."

☐ Short-term stress is good for you, and crucial to human survival.

☐ Chronic stress can lead to burnout, causing mental and physical damage.

☐ Stress and burnout are not the same. However, constant, recurring stress can lead to burnout.

☐ The negative, long-term effects of burnout include unhealthy physical and mental changes.

☐ The effects of long-term burnout can be treated successfully.

☐ Burnout lowers your body's natural defense system, meaning you are more susceptible to infection, illness and disease.

☐ One cause of burnout is when you feel like you lack any control in your life.

☐ A constant overload or overwork in your career or personal life can lead to burnout

☐ When you feel as if you don't "belong" to anything or any group, you could be experiencing the first stages of burnout

☐ A lack of satisfaction or personal/career rewards and appreciation is a sign that burnout could be right around the corner

☐ When you perceive that you are constantly unfairly treated, whether right or wrong, you are a prime candidate for burnout

☐ Avoiding burnout means exercising regularly, getting lots of sleep and staying hydrated

☐ Eat fewer processed foods, sweets, fried foods and anything that comes in a box, wrapper, can or package. These unhealthy foods cause physical stress.

☐ Eat more vegetables, fruits, berries and nuts, healthy food which lowers your natural stress levels.

☐ Stay away from stressful environments.

☐ Human beings are naturally social animals. Spend time with people who think the way you do, and loved ones who can offer support.

☐ Practicing meditation, aromatherapy, acupuncture and deep breathing techniques can prevent and treat burnout.

☐ Uncertainty leads to stress. Too much stress leads to burnout. Schedule your life, and then follow the schedule that you developed.

Some symptoms of burnout include ...

☐ Lack of motivation

☐ Withdrawing from society, and your responsibilities

☐ Frequent headaches

☐ Chronic muscle aches and back pain

☐ You feel alone in the world

☐ You are constantly tired and exhausted

☐ You feel there's nothing positive in the world or in your life

☐ You are sick all the time

☐ You frequently turn to alcohol, food and/or drugs as a treatment for the problems in your life

☐ You are never happy

☐ Nothing you ever do is good enough

☐ You experience a constant feeling of failure and self-doubt

☐ A recent change in your appetite and/or sleep habits that is drastic in nature

Final Thoughts

Stress is often a sign you have "too much on your plate". That saying is used to illustrate the fact that someone has more responsibilities, tasks and other commitments than they can handle. When this situation persists, this chronic stress, and your body's response to it, can lead you to feeling burned out altogether, and incapable of dealing with your normal, day-to-day life.

Prioritize, Prioritize, Prioritize

When you have too many commitments to keep up with, it is only natural to feel a sense of failure or depression when responsibilities are not handled. This is a sign that you are a responsible person. You have made commitments or had tasks handed down to you, and you work very hard to accomplish all of them.

Sometimes though, there don't seem to be enough hours in the day. Your personal and business responsibilities, as well as social activities, seem to pile up one on another until you experience constant stress, rather than a sense of accomplishment.

This is a sign you need to prioritize your world, and stop saying "yes" every time you are asked to help out.

What is really, truly important in your life? Ask yourself this question about your job, family, and yourself. Be very honest here. Understanding what **needs** to be done, and what you **want** to get done, as well as what you should **ignore**, helps you plan your day so that your most important responsibilities are handled first.

Take a Look at Your To-Do List

Write down everything you need to accomplish today, this week, this month and this year. Without writing it down, and simply relying on your memory, doesn't always work. Once you have your to-do list in front of you, circle or check those activities which only take a few minutes to finish.

Your list of responsibilities for today may have 15 items. Taken as a whole, that list can look pretty daunting. You are thinking about every task and commitment at the same time, but you can't accomplish more than one thing at a time.

Look at each item on your to do list individually. By grouping together those responsibilities which can be completed in a few minutes each, and then attacking them accordingly, you can often knock out a large part of your responsibilities in a short period of time.

Make Time for Yourself

If you are burned-out you can't help anyone, including yourself. Clear time in your schedule each day for "me" activities. You may be surprised that by making time for yourself throughout your busy schedule, you are more productive, and capable of accomplishing all of your scheduled activities.

Other Health and Fitness Books by This Author

If you would like to read more about Senior Health and Fitness, here is a list of the titles, CreateSpace links and descriptions:

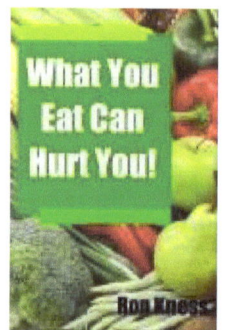

What You Eat Can Hurt You

Do you know that certain foods increase your risk for inflammation, disease and illness? It's true! And certain foods can help cure and heal you if you do get sick. Knowing which foods to eat and which ones to avoid empowers you to manage your own health.

https://www.createspace.com/4963196

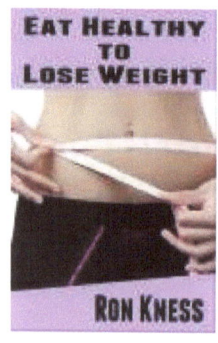

Eat Healthy to Lose Weight

As you read through our book, we show you which foods you should and should not be eating to reach your weight loss goal, along with discussing how to maintain your weight loss and stay within a few pounds of your goal weight. Banish the weight you keep gaining back each time by learning how to live a healthy lifestyle.

https://www.createspace.com/4962939

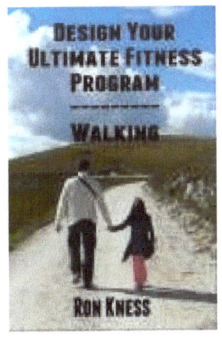

Design Your Ultimate Fitness Program - Walking

In my book Design Your Ultimate Fitness Program – Walking, we discuss the considerations that need to be made when designing a custom walking program, along with:

• Equipment needed
• Wearable technology you can use to track your walking
• And how to make walking more challenging

https://www.createspace.com/5252272

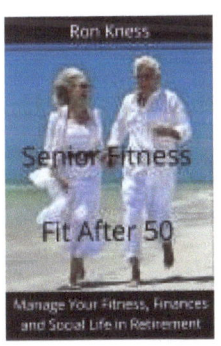

Senior Fitness – Fit After 50: Learn How to Manage Your Fitness, Finances and Social Life in Retirement

Inside you will discover answers to your most pressing questions:
• What do I need to know about downsizing my home?
• What are the best tips for staying healthy as you approach your 50's?
• When should I start planning for retirement?
• I am worried about being lonely once I retire, do others feel the same?
• Is it worthwhile to carry two homes during retirement?
And more...

https://www.createspace.com/5474751

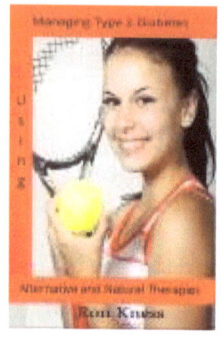

Managing Type 2 Diabetes Using Alternative And Natural Therapies

While Type 2 diabetes can be managed medically, there are many alternative natural and holistic methods of therapy and treatment that can further enhance quality of life and minimize the effects of this disease. In this book, I discuss 12 different types, including yoga, reflexology and acupuncture to name just three.

https://www.createspace.com/5401244

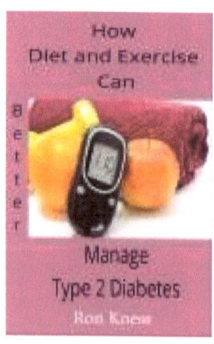

How Diet and Exercise Can Better Manage Type 2 Diabetes

Of the different types of diabetes, only Type 2 can be reversed. In my book How Diet and Exercise Can Better Manage Type 2 Diabetes, we reveal the three things you can do to best manage your disease, including:
• Diet
• Exercise
• Weight management

https://www.createspace.com/5404845

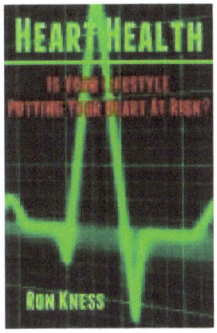

Heart Health: Is Your Lifestyle Putting Your Heart at Risk?

In my ebook Is Your Lifestyle Putting Your Heart At Risk? we discuss the six greatest risks to your heart and the lifestyle changes you can make to mitigate them.

https://www.createspace.com/5464020

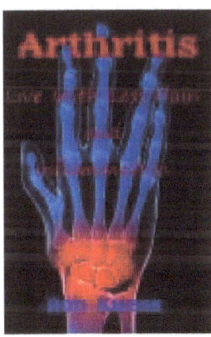

Arthritis – Live Wth Less Pain and Inflammation: Tips and Techniques You Can Use to Lessen the Pain and Inflammation

Discover Simple Tips & Information That Will Help Reduce The Painful Symptoms Of Arthritis!

You learn things like:
• Simple and effective information that will help you manage the pain and inflammation that comes along with arthritis, so that you can live an active, full life without debilitating pain.
• The different types of arthritis, their symptoms and how to alleviate their painful side effects.
• The pros and cons of over-the-counter arthritis medications, plus simple tips that will help you know how to choose the right supplements.
• Free, yet effective ways to get relief from arthritis

pain and inflammation, so you don't have to suffer anymore.

the effects arthritis can have significant impact on your physical and mental well-being, but this books shows you how to overcome its painful symptoms and live life relatively pain free.

https://www.createspace.com/5457441

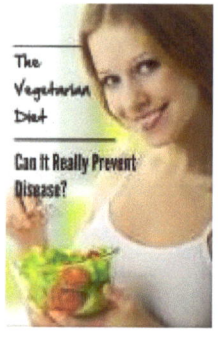

The Vegetarian Diet – Can It Really Prevent Disease?

Is a vegetarian diet right for you? Multiple studies have shown over and over that a vegetarian diet goes along way in preventing certain chronic diseases, such as:

• Heart Disease
• Cancer
• Diverticulitis
• Type 2 Diabetes
• Hypertension
• Obesity
• Kidney Failure

https://www.createspace.com/5519874

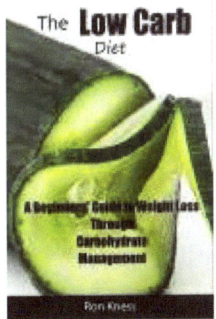

The Low Carb Diet: A Beginner's Guide to Weight Loss Through Carbohydrate Management

In my book "The Low-Carb Diet – A Beginners' Guide to Weight Loss Through Carbohydrate Management", I reveal a successful method of losing weight based in part on the amount and type of carbohydrates you consume.

https://www.createspace.com/5416348

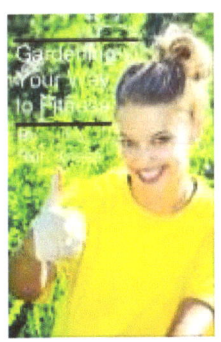

Gardening Your Way to Fitness: The Fun Way to Get Fit and Provide Beauty and Healthful Bounty for Your Family

The gym is a great place to stay fit during the colder seasons, but once the temperature turns warmer you want to spend more time outside. Plus, you'll have the benefit of fresh wholesome produce to enjoy by growing vegetables in your backyard garden.

https://www.createspace.com/5459564

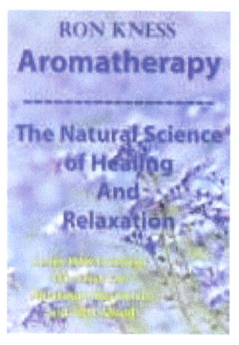

[Aromatherapy - The Science of Healing and Relaxation: Learn How Essential Oils Elicit The Relaxation Response And Alter Mood](#)

In my book Aromatherapy – The Science of Healing and Relaxation, we reveal the natural holistics methods you can use to heal the body from certain medical issues and to relive stress through relaxation. In particular we talk about:

• Aromatherapy - what it is and how it works

• Essential Oils – how the effects of certain aromas differs from others

• Recipes – how to make your own essential oil combinations

https://www.createspace.com/5714434

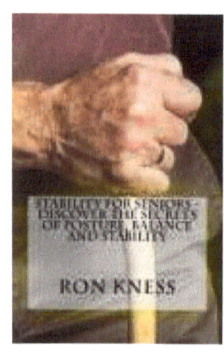

[Stability for Seniors: Discover the Secrets of Posture, Balance and Stability](#)

Many people sacrifice their health in pursuit of their career. They are so busy making a living that they neglect to make a life. The excuse that they do not have time to exercise is tossed about so frequently that they end up letting their health and fitness slide.

If you are not regularly active, you will have muscular atrophy over time.

Your flexibility will decrease. Your core strength will diminish. As time progresses, you will be less limber and more rigid.

This is exactly how people age poorly. It's a process that has snowballed over time.

Only with regular exercise and a healthy diet can you have a body that is fit and has the ability to almost reverse aging.

If you have neglected your health for years and life seems to be a chore now because you can't get around without assistance, do not feel dejected.

You can remedy the situation. You can restore the strength, balance and stamina that you have lost. It is never too late to become what you might have been.

This guide will show you exactly what you need to do to restore your balance, strengthen your core and give you the ability to live life to its fullest. Read how ...

https://www.createspace.com/6096479

About the Author

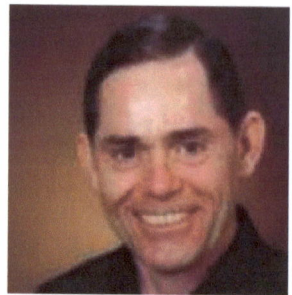

I grew up in Central Minnesota, where my parents owned and operated a fishing resort. Once out of high school I tried a couple of semesters of college, only to quit halfway through the Spring term; I decided at that time that college wasn't for me.

Then I decided to follow my father's previous occupation as an auto mechanic. I graduated from a two-year of vocational training course and worked as a mechanic for five years. While in vocational training, I decided to join the National Guard where I eventually ended up working full-time for 32 years.

So how does all of this relate to writing? In one of my leadership schools, the instructor, who was an English teacher at a juvenile detention center, presented writing to me in a whole new way - a way that started to develop my interest in working with words.

I eventually went back to college on the GI Bill while I was working and earned my Bachelor's degree in Business Administration.

Taking a class or two per semester at night and on weekends took me seven years to complete my degree.

Fast forward about 40 years and I now have published over 75 books on Amazon for Kindle, CreateSpace and other publishing platforms.

Besides my own writing, I also ghostwrite ebooks, reports, articles, blogs and do Kindle conversions for clients on a variety of topics.

Today my wife and I are retired from our careers and live in Gold Canyon, AZ. I now write as a retirement business where you'll find me happily sitting in my office typing away on my laptop as I work on my next book or ghostwriting project . . . that is if we are not traveling on a cruise ship - our new-found mode of travel.

www.ingramcontent.com/pod-product-compliance
Lightning Source LLC
Chambersburg PA
CBHW050830290526
45792CB00001B/340